Chapter 1: The Allure of Hollywood Skincare

The Glamour of the Red Carpet

The red carpet is often viewed as the pinnacle of glamour and celebrity culture, where stars strut in designer gowns and bespoke suits, capturing the attention of the world. However, this dazzling display is not merely about fashion; it is also a showcase for impeccable skin. Behind the scenes, celebrities and their teams invest significant time and resources into skincare regimens that ensure they look their best under the harsh glare of camera lights. The pursuit of a flawless complexion is a well-guarded secret that combines cutting-edge products and age-old techniques, all tailored to meet the intense demands of public appearances.

One of the most important aspects of red carpet preparation is the pre-event skincare routine. Celebrities often consult with top dermatologists and estheticians who provide tailored treatments aimed at achieving radiant skin. These professionals utilize advanced technologies like LED therapy, chemical peels, and microdermabrasion to refine the skin's texture and tone. These treatments are designed to address specific concerns such as acne, pigmentation, and signs of aging, ensuring that the star's skin not only looks good but feels healthy and rejuvenated. The synergy between professional skincare and at-home routines creates a powerful regimen that many celebrities swear by.

Another key element behind the glamour of the red carpet is the use of high-quality skincare products infused with unique ingredients. Many stars rely on serums and moisturizers that feature powerful compounds like hyaluronic acid, peptides, and antioxidants. These ingredients work together to hydrate, plump, and protect the skin, providing a dewy glow that is essential for high-definition cameras. Additionally, some celebrities turn to lesser-known ingredients, such as snail mucin or caviar extract, which are rumored to provide extraordinary benefits. The allure of these exotic components adds an element of mystique, further enhancing the fascination surrounding the red carpet.

Makeup artists play a crucial role in transforming the skincare foundation into a breathtaking final look. They often incorporate skincare-infused makeup products that complement the rigorous skincare routines. These products not only enhance the appearance of the skin but also nourish it throughout the event. Techniques such as layering primers, using luminous foundations, and setting sprays help achieve an ethereal glow that captures the essence of Hollywood glamour. The collaboration between skincare and makeup is a delicate balance, perfected through experience and innovation, contributing to the overall aesthetic that dazzles onlookers.

The impact of the red carpet extends far beyond the event itself; it influences trends and standards in the beauty industry. Many consumers aspire to replicate the looks seen on their favorite celebrities, leading to increased interest in high-performance skincare products and treatments. As the public becomes more aware of the importance of maintaining healthy skin, the secrets behind the glamour of the red carpet are increasingly revealed. This shift encourages a broader conversation about skincare, emphasizing that beauty is not merely superficial but a reflection of self-care, health, and confidence.

Why Skincare Matters in the Spotlight

In the glitzy world of Hollywood, where appearances are paramount, skincare often takes center stage. The entertainment industry thrives on visual aesthetics, making it essential for actors, actresses, and influencers to maintain flawless skin. This necessity has led to a growing awareness of skincare, not just as a routine but as a crucial aspect of one's public persona. The pressure to look impeccable is immense, driving many in the industry to invest substantial time and resources into their skincare regimens. Understanding why skincare matters in this spotlight can shed light on its broader implications for both celebrities and their audiences.

The quest for beautiful skin often leads to the exploration of unique and sometimes unconventional ingredients that are not widely known outside of Hollywood. Many celebrities turn to skincare products that feature rare botanicals, exotic oils, and cutting-edge formulations. These ingredients frequently become trends, inspiring fans to seek out the same products in hopes of achieving a similar glow. The influence of Hollywood on skincare is profound, as it not only shapes consumer behavior but also drives innovation within the skincare industry itself, pushing brands to develop new solutions that meet the demands of high-profile clients.

Moreover, the importance of skincare in Hollywood extends beyond mere appearance; it is also tied to self-confidence and mental well-being. For many in the industry, a well-crafted skincare routine serves as a form of self-care, providing a moment of tranquility amidst the chaos of fame. This practice is often shared with fans, reinforcing the idea that taking care of one's skin is not just about looking good but also about feeling good. The dialogue surrounding skincare has evolved, encouraging a more holistic view of beauty that encompasses both physical and emotional health.

As the public becomes increasingly aware of the secrets behind celebrity skincare, the demand for transparency rises. Fans want to know the ingredients that contribute to their favorite stars' radiant complexions. This shift has prompted brands to disclose more about their products and even collaborate with celebrities to create lines that resonate with their audience. The spotlight on skincare ingredients has led to a more educated consumer base, which is eager to learn about the benefits and origins of the products they use. This trend is reshaping the skincare market, prioritizing quality and efficacy over mere celebrity endorsement.

Ultimately, skincare in Hollywood serves as a powerful reminder of the relationship between beauty, health, and self-expression. The pursuit of skincare excellence is not solely about aesthetics; it reflects a deeper understanding of personal care and the desire for authenticity in an often superficial industry. As celebrities continue to share their skincare journeys, they influence a culture that values self-care and promotes the idea that everyone deserves to shine in their own right. This evolving narrative underscores the significance of skincare, making it a vital topic in discussions about beauty and wellness in the modern age.

Chapter 2: The Ingredients Behind the Glow

Rare Oils and Their Benefits

Rare oils have captivated the beauty industry, especially in Hollywood, where the allure of youthful, radiant skin is paramount. These oils, often sourced from remote corners of the globe, possess unique properties that set them apart from more common skincare ingredients. Their rich compositions and potential benefits are drawing attention from celebrities and beauty aficionados alike, eager to unlock the secrets behind their glowing complexions. From ancient traditions to modern formulations, rare oils are becoming essential in the quest for flawless skin.

One of the most notable rare oils is Marula oil, derived from the nuts of the Marula tree found in Southern Africa. This oil is packed with antioxidants, essential fatty acids, and vitamins C and E, making it a powerhouse for hydration and nourishment. Its lightweight texture absorbs quickly, making it ideal for all skin types. Marula oil not only helps to lock in moisture but also improves skin elasticity, reduces the appearance of fine lines, and provides a natural glow. This oil has become a staple in many Hollywood skincare routines, as it leaves the skin feeling soft and radiant without a greasy residue.

Another gem in the world of rare oils is Prickly Pear Seed Oil, also known as Barbary Fig oil. Extracted from the seeds of the prickly pear cactus, this oil is rich in vitamin E and essential fatty acids, which are known for their ability to restore skin elasticity and promote healing. Prickly Pear Seed Oil is especially beneficial for sensitive or inflamed skin, as it has anti-inflammatory properties that can soothe irritation and redness. Its high antioxidant content helps to combat free radicals, making it a powerful ally in preventing premature aging. Celebrities often turn to this oil for its ability to provide deep hydration while minimizing the appearance of pores.

Kukui Nut Oil, native to Hawaii, is another rare oil making waves in the skincare world. Renowned for its moisturizing properties, Kukui Nut Oil is rich in omega-3 and omega-6 fatty acids, which help to repair the skin's barrier and maintain hydration. This oil is particularly beneficial for dry or damaged skin, as it aids in healing and rejuvenation. Kukui Nut Oil absorbs quickly and leaves no greasy residue, making it suitable for daily use. Its natural ability to protect against environmental stressors has made it a favorite among Hollywood stars who need to keep their skin looking its best under harsh studio lights and outdoor shoots.

Lastly, Sea Buckthorn Oil, derived from the berries of the sea buckthorn plant, is celebrated for its wealth of nutrients, including vitamins A, C, and E, as well as a variety of antioxidants. This oil is known for its remarkable ability to promote skin regeneration and repair, making it an excellent option for those dealing with scarring or sun damage. Sea Buckthorn Oil also supports skin elasticity and hydration, which is crucial for maintaining a youthful appearance. Its unique blend of fatty acids and vitamins has garnered attention from top dermatologists and skincare experts, leading to its inclusion in high-end Hollywood skincare products aimed at achieving that coveted glow.

These rare oils not only enhance the efficacy of skincare routines but also symbolize the innovative spirit of the beauty industry. As Hollywood continues to embrace natural and effective ingredients, these oils stand out as luxurious yet potent solutions for achieving healthy, radiant skin. Exploring the benefits of these rare oils reveals the hidden secrets that contribute to the timeless beauty and allure of Hollywood icons.

Ancient Herbs and Modern Science

Ancient herbal remedies have been utilized for centuries across various cultures, revered for their healing properties and ability to enhance beauty. In the context of skincare, many of these herbs have gained renewed interest in modern science, revealing their potential to address contemporary skin concerns. Ingredients like aloe vera, calendula, and ginseng are not merely relics of the past; they are at the forefront of current skincare research, bridging the gap between traditional wisdom and scientific validation.

Aloe vera, often dubbed the "plant of immortality," has been used since ancient Egypt for its soothing and hydrating properties. Modern studies have confirmed its effectiveness in treating burns, wounds, and even acne, showcasing its versatility. Aloe vera is rich in vitamins, minerals, and antioxidants, making it an ideal ingredient for Hollywood's elite who seek to maintain a youthful glow. Its ability to promote skin healing and reduce inflammation aligns well with the fast-paced lifestyle of many in the entertainment industry, where the pressure to look flawless is ever-present.

Another ancient herb, calendula, has been cherished for its anti-inflammatory and antimicrobial properties. Historical records trace its use back to the Romans, who valued calendula for its ability to heal wounds and soothe skin irritations. Recent scientific explorations have validated these claims, revealing calendula's potential in promoting collagen synthesis and enhancing skin elasticity. This has made it a favored ingredient among skincare formulators in Hollywood, who harness its benefits to create products that address the signs of aging while ensuring skin remains resilient and vibrant.

Ginseng, a staple in traditional Asian medicine, is celebrated for its adaptogenic qualities and ability to rejuvenate the skin. Research has shown that ginseng extracts can improve skin hydration, reduce the appearance of fine lines, and enhance overall skin tone. As Hollywood stars look for ways to combat the effects of stress and environmental damage, ginseng-infused products have emerged as a popular choice. Its reputation for boosting energy and vitality translates well into skincare, aligning with the desire for a radiant complexion that reflects a healthy lifestyle.

Integrating these ancient herbs into modern skincare formulations exemplifies a growing trend in the beauty industry that values both heritage and innovation. As consumers become more aware of the origins of their skincare products, the demand for natural ingredients has surged. Hollywood's secret skincare formulations often draw inspiration from these time-honored herbs, combining them with cutting-edge technology to create effective and luxurious products. This fusion not only honors traditional practices but also highlights the importance of scientific validation, ensuring that the secrets behind the glow are both natural and effective.

Chapter 3: Celebrity Favorites

The Go-To Products of A-List Stars

The world of Hollywood is often synonymous with glamour, but behind the radiant skin of A-list stars lies a carefully curated selection of skincare products. These celebrities frequently rely on a combination of high-end brands and niche products that capitalize on unique ingredients. Understanding the go-to products of these stars offers insight into the secrets of achieving that coveted glow. From serums that promise to hydrate to masks that rejuvenate, these items are staples in the beauty routines of those who often find themselves in the limelight.

One of the most notable products favored by A-listers is hyaluronic acid. Known for its incredible ability to retain moisture, this ingredient is found in many serums and moisturizers used by celebrities. Stars like Zendaya and Jennifer Aniston have been vocal about their love for hyaluronic acid, often attributing their youthful appearance to its hydrating properties. It works by drawing in moisture from the environment, making it an essential component for anyone looking to maintain plump and dewy skin. These products are often layered into their routines, ensuring that hydration is maintained throughout the day.

Another essential in the kits of many Hollywood elites is vitamin C serum. This powerful antioxidant not only brightens the skin but also helps to combat the signs of aging by neutralizing free radicals. Celebrities such as Priyanka Chopra and Chris Hemsworth frequently mention their use of vitamin C in interviews, highlighting its ability to even out skin tone and enhance radiance. Many high-profile makeup artists recommend incorporating vitamin C into daily routines to create a perfect canvas for makeup application, ensuring that the skin looks vibrant and fresh.

For those seeking a quick and effective pick-me-up, sheet masks have become a favorite among stars. Products infused with ingredients like collagen, aloe vera, or green tea extract can provide an instant boost of hydration and nutrients. Celebrities like Kim Kardashian and Rihanna have been seen using sheet masks before public appearances to ensure their skin looks its best. These easy-to-use masks cater to various skin concerns, from dryness to dullness, making them a versatile addition to any skincare routine. The convenience of sheet masks also allows stars to pamper themselves even in the busiest of schedules.

Additionally, many A-list stars swear by the benefits of facial oils. These oils, which often contain a blend of nourishing ingredients like jojoba, rosehip, and argan oil, help to lock in moisture and provide a radiant finish. Stars like Emma Stone and Gigi Hadid have credited facial oils with transforming their skin, emphasizing their role in achieving a dewy, glowing complexion. These products are particularly popular among those with dry or combination skin types, as they can be layered over moisturizers or used alone for a lightweight yet hydrating finish.

In the ever-evolving landscape of beauty, the products favored by A-list stars reveal much about their skincare philosophies. From hyaluronic acid serums to revitalizing sheet masks, these items reflect a commitment to maintaining healthy skin amidst the pressures of public life. By incorporating these go-to products into their routines, celebrities not only enhance their appearance but also share valuable insights into achieving glowing skin. The secrets behind Hollywood's radiance may lie in these carefully chosen products, providing inspiration for anyone looking to elevate their skincare regimen.

Skincare Routines of Hollywood Icons

Skincare routines among Hollywood icons often reflect a blend of personal preferences, professional guidance, and access to exclusive products. Many celebrities emphasize the importance of consistency and tailoring routines to their skin types. For instance, stars like Jennifer Aniston advocate for a simple yet effective regimen that includes cleansing, moisturizing, and sun protection. Aniston has frequently spoken about her commitment to hydration and the use of high-quality moisturizers, which she believes are essential for maintaining a youthful appearance.

Another notable figure is Halle Berry, who attributes her radiant skin to a combination of healthy habits and premium skincare products. Berry is known to incorporate antioxidants into her routine, often using serums rich in vitamin C to combat oxidative stress from environmental factors. This approach not only enhances her skin's luminosity but also provides a protective barrier against free radicals. Her emphasis on a balanced diet further complements her skincare, showcasing the interconnectedness of nutrition and skin health.

Angelina Jolie's skincare regimen includes a focus on natural and organic products, reflecting her commitment to sustainability. Jolie often opts for skincare lines that prioritize clean ingredients, steering clear of harsh chemicals. Her routine usually features gentle cleansers, nourishing oils, and hydrating masks. This choice emphasizes the rising trend among Hollywood stars to seek out products that are not only effective but also environmentally friendly, aligning with a broader movement towards conscious consumerism in the beauty industry.

The influence of professional dermatologists and estheticians cannot be understated in the skincare routines of Hollywood elites. Many stars, such as Kim Kardashian, regularly consult with skin experts who tailor treatments to their specific needs. Kardashian's routine often includes chemical peels and laser treatments, which help maintain her skin's texture and clarity. This highlights the importance of professional intervention in achieving and sustaining flawless skin, particularly in an industry where appearance is paramount.

In addition to their individual routines, Hollywood icons often share a common secret: the use of innovative ingredients that may not be widely accessible. Ingredients like snail mucin, derived from the secretion of snails, and various plant stem cells have gained popularity among celebrities for their remarkable regenerative properties. These components are often incorporated into high-end skincare lines that promise to deliver transformative results. By embracing such unique ingredients, Hollywood stars not only enhance their skin but also set trends that influence skincare enthusiasts around the globe.

Chapter 4: The Science of Skincare

Understanding Active Ingredients

Active ingredients are the cornerstone of any effective skincare regimen, particularly in the high-stakes world of Hollywood. These components are scientifically formulated to deliver specific benefits, addressing issues such as aging, pigmentation, and hydration. Understanding active ingredients is essential for anyone looking to achieve glowing skin, as they play a pivotal role in determining the efficacy of products. In Hollywood, where flawless skin is often under the spotlight, the selection and application of active ingredients are approached with precision and care.

Among the most recognized active ingredients are retinoids, which derive from vitamin A. Retinoids are celebrated for their ability to promote cell turnover, diminish fine lines, and enhance skin texture. In the fast-paced environment of Hollywood, where makeup artists frequently apply heavy cosmetics, retinoids help to maintain skin health by preventing clogged pores and reducing acne outbreaks. Celebrities often incorporate retinoids into their nighttime skincare routines to ensure their skin remains luminous and camera-ready.

Another crucial category of active ingredients includes antioxidants, such as vitamin C and E. These compounds combat oxidative stress caused by environmental factors like pollution and UV radiation, which can accelerate skin aging. In Hollywood, where outdoor events and red carpets expose skin to harsh elements, the use of antioxidants is paramount. They not only help to protect the skin but also brighten the complexion, making them a favorite among actors and actresses who need to look their best at all times.

Peptides are gaining traction in the skincare routines of Hollywood's elite. These small chains of amino acids are vital for building proteins like collagen and elastin, which are essential for maintaining skin firmness and elasticity. As the demand for youthful skin grows, celebrities are increasingly turning to peptide-infused products to combat sagging and enhance overall skin resilience. The strategic use of peptides in both daily skincare and professional treatments reflects a sophisticated understanding of skin biology, aligning perfectly with the demands of the entertainment industry.

Finally, hyaluronic acid stands out as a superstar active ingredient known for its remarkable hydrating properties. Capable of holding up to 1,000 times its weight in water, hyaluronic acid helps to maintain skin moisture levels, promoting a plump and youthful appearance. In Hollywood, where the pressure to maintain perfect skin can lead to dryness from makeup and environmental stressors, hyaluronic acid serves as a hydration hero. Its inclusion in serums and moisturizers is a common practice among those in the industry, ensuring that their skin remains well-hydrated and radiant, even under the harshest conditions. Understanding these active ingredients not only empowers consumers to make informed choices but also reveals the meticulous care that goes into achieving the enviable skin seen on Hollywood's brightest stars.

The Role of pH in Skincare

The pH level of a product plays a crucial role in skincare, influencing how effectively it interacts with the skin. The pH scale ranges from 0 to 14, with 7 being neutral. Skin is naturally slightly acidic, typically ranging from 4.5 to 5.5, which helps maintain the skin's barrier function and overall health. When skincare products are formulated to match the skin's natural pH, they can enhance the skin's ability to absorb beneficial ingredients, promote healing, and reduce irritation. Conversely, products with an inappropriate pH can disrupt this balance, leading to various skin issues such as dryness, irritation, and even acne.

In Hollywood, where the quest for flawless skin is paramount, many celebrities and skincare experts emphasize the importance of pH-balanced products. They often seek out formulations that align with their skin's natural acidity to achieve a radiant complexion. Ingredients like hyaluronic acid and lactic acid are popular in this realm, as they not only hydrate but also help maintain an optimal pH level. The right balance can also assist in preventing the overgrowth of harmful bacteria, ensuring that the skin remains healthy and glowing.

Additionally, understanding pH is essential when introducing new products into a skincare routine. For instance, combining products with significantly different pH levels can lead to an unwanted reaction. Acidic products might neutralize the effects of more alkaline treatments, diminishing their efficacy. This is particularly crucial for those using active ingredients such as retinoids or acids, which require specific pH levels to perform optimally. Celebrities often consult with skincare professionals to curate a regimen that respects the pH balance for maximum results.

Moreover, the impact of pH extends beyond just product formulation. Environmental factors such as pollution, diet, and lifestyle can also influence the skin's acidity. For example, a diet high in sugar and processed foods can lead to an increase in skin pH, potentially resulting in breakouts and dullness. Hollywood stars frequently advocate for a holistic approach to skincare, emphasizing that what goes into the body is just as important as what is applied topically. This awareness helps them maintain their skin's health and appearance over time.

Ultimately, the role of pH in skincare is a multifaceted aspect that deserves attention. As the industry continues to evolve, the integration of pH awareness into product development and skincare routines will likely become more prevalent. Those seeking Hollywood-worthy skin can benefit from understanding the significance of pH and choosing products that support their skin's natural balance, unlocking the secrets to achieving that coveted glow.

Chapter 5: DIY Secrets from Hollywood

At-Home Treatments of the Stars

At-home treatments have become a staple in Hollywood, where the desire for glowing skin is often paired with busy schedules and high expectations. Celebrities frequently turn to simple yet effective remedies that can be easily integrated into their daily routines. These treatments often draw from natural ingredients and time-tested techniques, showcasing how stars maintain their radiant appearances without always relying on expensive salon visits or invasive procedures.

One of the most popular at-home treatments among A-listers is the use of honey and avocado masks. Honey, known for its antibacterial properties, not only helps in clearing blemishes but also acts as a natural moisturizer. When combined with avocado, which is rich in healthy fats and vitamins, this mask becomes a nourishing powerhouse. Many celebrities swear by this duo, applying it weekly to keep their skin hydrated and supple, while also ensuring a radiant glow for those red carpet events.

Another favored method is the incorporation of essential oils into skincare routines. Stars like Miranda Kerr and Emma Watson have been advocates for using oils such as rosehip and tea tree. Rosehip oil is celebrated for its ability to reduce scars and fine lines, while tea tree oil is a go-to for combating acne. By diluting these oils with a carrier oil, celebrities can create a personalized treatment that addresses their specific skin concerns, making it not only effective but also a luxurious experience.

Exfoliation is key for maintaining smooth skin, and many Hollywood figures have embraced DIY scrubs made from common kitchen ingredients. A simple scrub using coffee grounds and coconut oil can invigorate the skin, promoting circulation while sloughing away dead skin cells. This treatment is particularly popular among stars preparing for big events, as it leaves their skin looking fresh and vibrant. Regular exfoliation ensures that makeup applies smoothly, enhancing the overall glam look that is essential for film premieres and awards shows.

Finally, hydration is a crucial component of any at-home skincare regimen, and celebrities often turn to infused water to keep their skin glowing from the inside out. Infusing water with ingredients like cucumber, lemon, and mint not only makes it refreshing but also packs a punch of antioxidants and vitamins. Stars often share their hydration hacks on social media, emphasizing the importance of drinking plenty of water for a clear complexion. This simple yet effective practice underscores the idea that maintaining beautiful skin can be achieved through accessible means that fit seamlessly into a busy lifestyle.

Kitchen Ingredients for Radiant Skin

In the quest for radiant skin, many individuals often overlook the treasures that lie within their own kitchens. Everyday ingredients, commonly found in your pantry or refrigerator, can offer significant benefits for skin health and appearance. From fruits and vegetables to oils and spices, these natural components can provide the nourishment and hydration that contribute to a glowing complexion. By incorporating these kitchen staples into your skincare routine, you can unlock the secrets to achieving that coveted Hollywood glow, all while avoiding synthetic chemicals and expensive products.

Coconut oil is one such ingredient that has gained popularity not just in the culinary world but also in skincare. Rich in fatty acids, it acts as a natural moisturizer, helping to hydrate the skin and lock in moisture. Its antibacterial properties can help combat acne, making it a versatile option for various skin types. Simply applying a small amount to your face or using it as a base for a DIY scrub can provide immediate benefits. Additionally, its lightweight texture makes it suitable for daily use, providing a luminous finish without clogging pores.

Another powerhouse ingredient is honey, a staple in many kitchens known for its natural humectant properties. Honey draws moisture from the environment into the skin, making it an excellent choice for keeping the skin hydrated and plump. Its antioxidant and anti-inflammatory properties can help soothe irritated skin and reduce redness. Applying honey as a mask or mixing it with other ingredients like yogurt or oatmeal can create a nourishing treatment that enhances the skin's natural radiance, offering a spa-like experience at home.

Fruits such as avocados and bananas are also rich in vitamins and healthy fats that can improve skin texture and appearance. Avocados, packed with vitamins E and C, help protect the skin from oxidative stress while providing deep hydration. When mashed and applied as a mask, they can leave the skin feeling soft and rejuvenated. Bananas, on the other hand, contain potassium and vitamins that can help soothe and moisturize the skin. Their natural exfoliating properties make them an ideal ingredient for homemade treatments that promote a brighter complexion.

Spices like turmeric and cinnamon are not just flavor enhancers but also offer significant skincare benefits. Turmeric is renowned for its anti-inflammatory and antiseptic properties, making it a fantastic option for reducing breakouts and evening skin tone. When mixed with yogurt or honey, it forms a powerful mask that can brighten the skin and combat dullness. Cinnamon, with its ability to stimulate blood flow, can promote a healthy glow and improve overall skin texture. Incorporating these spices into your skincare routine can provide a natural boost to your skin's radiance and vitality.

Incorporating these kitchen ingredients into your skincare regimen not only promotes healthy and radiant skin but also empowers individuals to take control of their beauty routines. By utilizing accessible and natural components, you can achieve results similar to those sought after in Hollywood while keeping your routine simple and sustainable. The next time you're in your kitchen, consider the potential of these ingredients; they may just hold the key to unlocking your most luminous skin yet.

Chapter 6: Industry Insider Tips

The Role of Dermatologists in Hollywood

In Hollywood, where appearance often dictates success, dermatologists play a crucial role in maintaining the skin health of celebrities. With the industry's intense focus on physical beauty, these medical professionals are sought after for their expertise in preventing and treating skin issues that can arise from the pressures of fame. From acne and rosacea to the effects of aging, dermatologists provide tailored treatments that help stars look their best both on and off the screen. Their knowledge of skin conditions and the latest advancements in dermatological science is instrumental in creating personalized skincare regimens that enhance and protect the complexions of Hollywood's elite.

Dermatologists in Hollywood are not only focused on addressing existing skin problems but also on preventative care. Many celebrities visit dermatologists regularly to receive comprehensive skin assessments that identify potential issues before they become visible. This proactive approach often includes recommendations for at-home skincare routines that incorporate professional-grade products, which may contain unique and effective ingredients unknown to the general public. These tailored regimens can include everything from prescription-strength retinoids to advanced moisturizers designed specifically for the unique needs of high-profile clients.

In addition to traditional dermatological services, many Hollywood dermatologists specialize in cosmetic procedures that enhance a celebrity's appearance without sacrificing their natural beauty. Treatments such as chemical peels, laser therapy, and injectables like Botox and fillers have become commonplace among stars looking to rejuvenate their skin. Dermatologists in this niche use cutting-edge techniques and technology to ensure results are subtle yet effective, allowing their clients to maintain a youthful glow while minimizing downtime. The demand for such procedures has led to an increased emphasis on safety and efficacy, making it imperative for dermatologists to stay updated on the latest trends and research in cosmetic dermatology.

The relationship between dermatologists and their celebrity clients often goes beyond mere professional interaction. Many Hollywood stars form long-lasting partnerships with their dermatologists, who become trusted confidants in their skincare journeys. This bond can lead to exclusive insights into the skincare routines and ingredients that are effective for maintaining a flawless complexion under the scrutiny of cameras and public appearances. Dermatologists share their knowledge with clients, guiding them on how to select the right products and make informed choices that align with their skin type and lifestyle.

Finally, the influence of Hollywood dermatologists extends beyond their immediate clientele. Many of these professionals contribute to the broader skincare industry by developing their own product lines or collaborating with established brands to create innovative skincare solutions. Their firsthand experience with the unique needs of high-profile individuals allows them to craft formulations that can benefit a wider audience. As a result, the skincare secrets revealed by these dermatologists often become trends that shape consumer preferences and innovations within the market, demonstrating the profound impact that these specialists have on both individual and collective beauty standards.

Common Myths and Misconceptions

The world of skincare is rife with myths and misconceptions, particularly when it comes to the secrets that Hollywood stars swear by. One prevalent myth is that expensive skincare products are always more effective than their budget-friendly counterparts. While it is true that many high-end brands offer advanced formulations, there are numerous affordable products that contain equally effective ingredients. The efficacy of a skincare product often depends on its formulation and the specific needs of the skin rather than its price tag. Many celebrities endorse products that may carry a hefty price but often have accessible alternatives that deliver similar results.

Another common misconception is that natural ingredients are always the safest and most beneficial for the skin. While many natural components, such as aloe vera and coconut oil, provide significant advantages, they are not universally suitable for all skin types. Some individuals may experience allergic reactions or irritations from seemingly harmless ingredients. Additionally, synthetic ingredients can also be beneficial, as they often undergo rigorous testing and come with proven efficacy. Understanding one's skin type and conducting patch tests can help dispel the myth that natural is always better.

The belief that skincare routines need to be overly complicated is another widespread myth. Many assume that achieving glowing skin requires a lengthy regimen filled with numerous products. In reality, an effective skincare routine can be remarkably simple. A basic routine focusing on cleansing, moisturizing, and sun protection is often sufficient for most individuals. Celebrities often emphasize the importance of consistency over complexity, showcasing that a well-chosen set of products can yield impressive results without overwhelming the user.

Additionally, there is a misconception surrounding the idea that celebrities have flawless skin due to their rigorous skincare routines alone. While it is true that many Hollywood stars invest time and effort into their skincare, genetics play a significant role in skin appearance. Factors such as diet, hydration, and lifestyle choices also greatly impact skin health. Many stars also rely on professional treatments that are not accessible to the general public, which can contribute to their seemingly perfect complexions. Acknowledging the blend of genetics and lifestyle choices helps demystify the allure of celebrity skin.

Lastly, the myth that skincare products work instantly is misleading. Many consumers expect immediate results from products, leading to disappointment when they do not see quick changes. In reality, effective skincare requires time and patience. Ingredients like retinoids, vitamin C, and hyaluronic acid can take weeks or even months to show noticeable improvements. Understanding that skincare is a long-term investment rather than a quick fix is essential for setting realistic expectations. This perspective allows individuals to appreciate the gradual transformation of their skin and encourages them to stick with routines that ultimately yield significant benefits.

Chapter 7: The Evolution of Skincare

Historical Practices in Hollywood

The historical practices in Hollywood regarding skincare have evolved significantly, shaped by cultural trends, technological advancements, and the ever-present desire for beauty and youth. In the early days of filmmaking, actors relied on basic skincare routines that often included natural ingredients such as olive oil, honey, and herbal infusions. These simple methods were born out of necessity and a lack of access to specialized products. Stars of the silent film era often faced the challenge of maintaining their appearance under harsh studio lights, which led them to experiment with various home remedies to protect their skin from damage.

As Hollywood transitioned into the Golden Age of cinema, the beauty industry began to flourish, leading to the emergence of iconic skincare products. The introduction of commercial cosmetics in the 1920s allowed actors to enhance their features on screen, but it also highlighted the importance of skincare as a foundation for makeup. Stars like Marilyn Monroe and Audrey Hepburn became known not just for their on-screen performances but also for their radiant complexions. Their skincare routines often included a mix of luxury creams and protective oils, laying the groundwork for the modern celebrity skincare regimen that prioritizes both prevention and enhancement.

In the 1950s and 1960s, Hollywood's beauty standards began to shift, influenced by the rise of youth culture and the countercultural movements of the time. This period saw an increased interest in natural beauty and organic ingredients, with celebrities advocating for simpler skincare practices. The use of vitamin E, aloe vera, and other botanicals became popular as actors sought to achieve a fresh, dewy look. This shift not only reflected changing societal values but also marked the beginning of a more holistic approach to skincare, one that acknowledged the importance of health and well-being.

The 1980s and 1990s brought about a technological revolution in skincare, with the introduction of innovative ingredients and formulations. Hollywood's elite began to embrace chemical peels, microdermabrasion, and other advanced treatments that promised to reverse the signs of aging. The influence of dermatologists and skincare professionals became more pronounced, with many celebrities collaborating with experts to develop personalized regimens. This era also saw the birth of the celebrity endorsement, as stars began to align themselves with specific brands and products, further shaping public perceptions of beauty and skincare.

Today, the legacy of historical skincare practices in Hollywood continues to influence the industry. The rise of social media has democratized access to beauty secrets, allowing influencers and celebrities to share their skincare routines with a global audience. As a result, there is a renewed interest in the ingredients that have stood the test of time, as well as a fascination with the innovative products that promise to deliver results. The blending of historical practices with modern science highlights the ongoing evolution of skincare, demonstrating that the quest for beauty is both a timeless pursuit and a reflection of contemporary values.

The Shift Towards Natural Ingredients

The beauty industry has witnessed a significant shift towards natural ingredients in recent years, particularly in Hollywood, where skincare trends often set the stage for broader consumer preferences. This transition is driven by increasing consumer awareness regarding the potential side effects of synthetic ingredients found in many mainstream products. As celebrities and influencers advocate for cleaner, more sustainable choices, natural ingredients have gained prominence. This movement reflects not only a desire for healthier skin but also a growing concern for environmental sustainability, urging brands to rethink their formulations.

Natural ingredients are often lauded for their effectiveness and gentleness on the skin. Many of these components, such as plant extracts, essential oils, and herbal infusions, have been used for centuries in traditional skincare practices. In Hollywood, where the pursuit of flawless skin is paramount, the use of these ingredients aligns with the desire for effective solutions without the harsh chemicals that can cause irritation or long-term damage. Products formulated with natural ingredients tend to be more compatible with various skin types, making them appealing to a diverse range of consumers seeking results without compromise.

The influence of celebrity endorsements cannot be overstated in this context. Many Hollywood stars have begun to champion brands that prioritize natural ingredients, sharing their personal skincare routines with their audiences. This visibility has propelled the popularity of clean beauty products, making them accessible and desirable. As more celebrities launch their own skincare lines featuring natural ingredients, they not only promote individual brands but also shift the overall narrative in the beauty industry towards a more holistic approach to skincare.

Moreover, the rise of social media has played a crucial role in this shift. Platforms like Instagram and TikTok serve as powerful tools for sharing skin care tips and product recommendations. Influencers and beauty gurus highlight the benefits of natural ingredients, often showcasing their effectiveness in achieving radiant skin. This digital landscape fosters a community where consumers can learn about the origins and benefits of these ingredients, further fueling the demand for products that are not only effective but also align with values of transparency and sustainability.

As the movement towards natural ingredients continues to gain momentum, the beauty industry is likely to see further innovation. Brands are now investing in research to discover new plant-based ingredients and sustainable sourcing methods. This evolution not only promises to enhance product efficacy but also ensures that consumers can feel good about their choices. In Hollywood and beyond, the embrace of natural ingredients represents a broader cultural shift toward wellness and authenticity, redefining beauty standards and encouraging a more mindful approach to skincare.

Chapter 8: The Future of Skincare

Trends to Watch in Hollywood

As Hollywood continues to evolve, several trends are emerging that significantly impact the skincare industry. One prominent trend is the increasing emphasis on clean and sustainable beauty products. Celebrities and influencers are advocating for transparency in ingredient sourcing and formulation. This shift is driven by a growing awareness of the environmental and health impacts of traditional cosmetics. Brands that prioritize eco-friendly practices and use natural, organic ingredients are gaining traction, appealing to both consumers and industry insiders. As this trend grows, expect to see a rise in products that are not only effective but also align with ethical standards.

Another trend gaining momentum is the integration of advanced technology in skincare. Innovations such as artificial intelligence and augmented reality are transforming how consumers engage with skincare products. For instance, apps that analyze skin conditions and suggest personalized skincare routines are becoming more popular. Additionally, brands are utilizing technology to enhance product formulations with cutting-edge ingredients that promise results. This fusion of technology and skincare is not just a passing fad; it represents a fundamental shift in how products are developed and marketed, particularly in the fast-paced Hollywood environment where appearance is paramount.

The rise of DIY skincare is also noteworthy as more consumers seek to create their own products at home. Influencers and beauty gurus are sharing recipes and tutorials that showcase how to use simple, natural ingredients to achieve glowing skin. This trend is partly fueled by the desire for customization and control over beauty regimens. In Hollywood, where unique looks are often celebrated, the ability to tailor skincare solutions is particularly appealing. As DIY skincare becomes mainstream, brands may respond by offering kits and ingredients for consumers to experiment with at home, merging convenience with creativity.

In addition, the wellness movement is influencing skincare trends in Hollywood. As the line between beauty and wellness continues to blur, consumers are increasingly seeking products that promote overall health rather than just aesthetic appeal. Ingredients known for their therapeutic benefits, such as adaptogens and probiotics, are making their way into skincare formulations. Celebrities are often at the forefront of this trend, endorsing products that not only enhance beauty but also support mental and physical well-being. As this trend gains traction, expect to see a surge in holistic approaches to skincare that prioritize health alongside beauty.

Lastly, inclusivity in beauty is becoming a significant focus in Hollywood. The industry is recognizing the importance of catering to diverse skin types and tones, leading to a broader range of products designed for all consumers. This shift is not only socially responsible but also commercially beneficial, as brands that embrace diversity can reach wider audiences and foster loyalty. As more celebrities and industry leaders advocate for inclusivity, the demand for products that address various skincare concerns across different demographics will continue to grow, reshaping the landscape of Hollywood skincare.

Innovations in Skincare Technology

Innovations in skincare technology have transformed the beauty industry, bringing groundbreaking solutions and products that cater to the unique needs of various skin types. In Hollywood, where flawless skin is often a prerequisite for success, the demand for advanced skincare is particularly high. This has led to a surge in research and development focused on creating effective formulations that not only enhance appearance but also promote long-term skin health. New technologies, such as nanotechnology and bioengineering, have enabled the delivery of active ingredients at a deeper level, maximizing their efficacy.

One of the most significant advancements in skincare technology is the use of personalized skincare solutions. Brands are increasingly leveraging artificial intelligence and data analytics to create customized products tailored to individual skin concerns. By analyzing factors such as skin type, environmental influences, and lifestyle habits, these innovative systems can recommend specific ingredients and formulations that are most effective for each user. This personalization trend resonates strongly in Hollywood, where celebrities seek products that address their unique skin challenges while ensuring optimal results.

Another notable innovation is the integration of biotechnology in skincare formulations. Ingredients derived from natural sources are being harnessed using advanced techniques that enhance their potency and stability. For instance, the use of probiotics and prebiotics in skincare products has gained traction, as these components help balance the skin's microbiome, leading to healthier and more resilient skin. Hollywood's elite have embraced these formulations, often featuring them in their daily routines to maintain their enviable glow.

Moreover, the rise of clean beauty has prompted brands to develop sustainable and eco-friendly products without compromising on effectiveness. Innovations in extraction methods and ingredient sourcing have led to the emergence of potent natural ingredients that provide similar, if not superior, results to traditional synthetic options. Many Hollywood stars advocate for these clean products, aligning their skincare choices with a growing consumer demand for transparency and ethical practices in the beauty industry.

Lastly, the incorporation of high-tech devices and tools has revolutionized skincare routines. At-home devices that utilize LED light therapy, ultrasonic waves, and microcurrent technology have become popular among skincare enthusiasts, including those in Hollywood. These tools enhance product absorption, stimulate collagen production, and improve skin texture, allowing users to achieve professional-grade results in the comfort of their homes. As technology continues to evolve, the future of skincare holds even more promise, with ongoing research suggesting that innovations will play a crucial role in redefining beauty standards and practices in Hollywood and beyond.

Chapter 9: Ethical and Sustainable Practices

The Push for Clean Beauty

The push for clean beauty has emerged as a significant movement within the cosmetics and skincare industry, particularly in Hollywood, where image and aesthetics play a critical role. This shift is driven by a growing awareness among consumers about the harmful effects of certain chemicals commonly found in beauty products. As celebrities and influencers increasingly advocate for transparency in ingredient sourcing and formulation, the clean beauty trend has gained momentum, prompting brands to reevaluate their practices and prioritize natural, non-toxic ingredients.

In Hollywood, where appearances are paramount, the demand for clean beauty products reflects a deeper cultural transformation. Many stars are now vocal proponents of using skincare and makeup that are not only effective but also safe for both the body and the environment. This advocacy has led to the rise of various clean beauty brands, many of which emphasize ethical sourcing, cruelty-free testing, and sustainable packaging. Consumers are increasingly looking for products that align with their values, seeking out brands that are committed to reducing their environmental footprint while delivering visible results.

Key ingredients in clean beauty products often include botanicals, essential oils, and plant-derived substances that offer nourishing benefits without harmful side effects. Hollywood's leading beauty experts and dermatologists have begun to highlight these ingredients, showcasing their efficacy in promoting healthy skin. This has led to a surge in interest surrounding products that harness the power of nature, such as hyaluronic acid derived from plant sources, or antioxidants sourced from fruits and herbs. The shift towards cleaner formulations not only enhances skin health but also promotes a holistic approach to beauty that resonates with consumers seeking authenticity.

The regulatory landscape surrounding cosmetic ingredients is also evolving, with increased scrutiny on the substances used in mainstream products. As consumers demand more transparency, brands are feeling the pressure to disclose their ingredient lists and the potential impact of these chemicals on health and the environment. This has prompted many companies to reformulate their products to eliminate harmful additives, such as parabens, sulfates, and synthetic fragrances. As a result, the clean beauty movement is not just a trend but a necessary response to a more informed consumer base that prioritizes safety and sustainability.

The future of clean beauty in Hollywood appears bright, as more celebrities and beauty influencers continue to champion the cause. This growing awareness is expected to lead to even more innovation in the industry, with brands exploring new, eco-friendly materials and sustainable practices. As Hollywood embraces the clean beauty ethos, it sets a powerful example for consumers everywhere, encouraging them to make informed choices about the products they use. Ultimately, the push for clean beauty represents a significant cultural shift towards prioritizing health, wellness, and environmental consciousness in the pursuit of beauty.

Celebrity Brands Leading the Change

In recent years, the intersection of celebrity culture and skincare has become increasingly pronounced, with numerous Hollywood stars launching their own brands. These celebrity-owned skincare lines often reflect a deep commitment to innovation and sustainability, showcasing unique formulations and ingredients that resonate with consumers. By leveraging their influence, these celebrities are not only promoting their products but also advocating for greater awareness about skincare and the importance of self-care in our daily routines.

One notable example is Rihanna's Fenty Skin, which has quickly gained a reputation for its inclusivity and effectiveness. The brand emphasizes clean ingredients and caters to a diverse audience, highlighting the importance of representation in beauty. Fenty Skin's formulations incorporate standout components like hyaluronic acid and niacinamide, promoting hydration and radiance for all skin types. By championing a message of inclusivity, Rihanna's brand leads the charge for a more holistic approach to skincare, encouraging individuals to embrace their unique beauty.

Similarly, actress Jessica Alba's Honest Beauty has made waves within the industry by focusing on transparency and ethical sourcing. The brand prides itself on using natural, non-toxic ingredients, appealing to consumers who are increasingly concerned about the safety and purity of the products they apply to their skin. With an array of skincare products that prioritize environmental sustainability, Honest Beauty represents a shift towards more mindful consumption in the beauty market. Alba's commitment to social responsibility has positioned her brand as a leader in the movement for cleaner, safer skincare products.

In addition to these specific brands, the phenomenon of celebrity collaborations with established skincare lines is also noteworthy. Collaborations often result in unique products that blend the celebrity's vision with the expertise of seasoned skincare professionals. These partnerships can lead to innovative formulations that leverage the latest advancements in skin science while also reflecting the personal care philosophies of the celebrities involved. This trend not only elevates the brands but also fosters a culture of creativity and experimentation within the skincare community.

Ultimately, celebrity brands are reshaping the skincare landscape by inspiring consumers to be more conscious of their choices. The influence of Hollywood stars extends beyond mere marketing; it encourages a dialogue about skincare that emphasizes the importance of quality ingredients and ethical practices. As these brands lead the charge towards innovation and sustainability, they are not just selling products but are also igniting a passion for skincare that prioritizes health, beauty, and individual expression. The impact of these celebrity-driven initiatives is paving the way for a new era in skincare, one that champions both efficacy and responsibility.

Chapter 10: Your Hollywood Routine

Creating a Personalized Skincare Regimen

Creating a personalized skincare regimen is essential for achieving healthy, glowing skin, especially when navigating the diverse and often overwhelming world of skincare products. The first step in this journey is understanding your skin type. Skin can generally be categorized into four types: oily, dry, combination, and sensitive. Each type has its own unique needs and requires specific ingredients to address its concerns. Oily skin, for instance, benefits from lightweight, oil-free products, while dry skin thrives on rich, hydrating formulas. Identifying your skin type will provide a foundation for building a regimen tailored to your specific needs.

Once you've determined your skin type, the next step is to assess your skin concerns. Common issues include acne, aging, hyperpigmentation, and dehydration. Each concern may require different active ingredients. For acne-prone skin, look for products with salicylic acid or benzoyl peroxide, while those dealing with signs of aging may benefit from retinoids and antioxidants. Hollywood's secret skincare ingredients often feature powerful botanicals and innovative compounds that target these specific issues. For example, the use of niacinamide in many high-end products can help reduce inflammation and improve skin texture, making it a favorite among A-list stars.

In addition to selecting the right ingredients, the order in which you apply your products plays a crucial role in their effectiveness. A well-structured skincare routine typically follows a specific sequence: cleanse, tone, treat, moisturize, and protect. Cleansing removes dirt and oil, while toners can help balance the skin's pH. Treatments, which include serums and targeted solutions, should be applied next to address specific concerns. A good moisturizer locks in hydration, and sunscreen is vital to protect the skin from harmful UV rays. Many Hollywood stars emphasize the importance of proper layering to maximize the benefits of skincare products.

Consistency is key to seeing results from your personalized skincare regimen. Establishing a daily routine that you can stick to will yield better long-term outcomes than sporadic use of products. Many celebrities adhere to strict skincare schedules, often incorporating both morning and evening routines. Evening regimens can be particularly beneficial as they allow the skin to recover and regenerate overnight. Keeping a skincare journal to track how your skin responds to different products can also be helpful in making necessary adjustments and ensuring you are on the right path.

Finally, it is essential to remember that everyone's skin is unique, and what works for one person may not work for another. It may take time to find the perfect combination of products and routines that suit your skin. Being patient and open to experimentation is part of the process. Moreover, seeking advice from skincare professionals or dermatologists can provide invaluable insights tailored specifically to your skin. By incorporating Hollywood's hidden skincare secrets and personalizing your approach, you can unveil your best skin yet.

Tips for Achieving That Hollywood Glow

Achieving that coveted Hollywood glow requires more than just good lighting; it starts with a solid skincare routine. One of the first tips is to establish a consistent cleansing ritual. Cleansing not only removes dirt and makeup but also prepares the skin to absorb the nourishing ingredients from serums and moisturizers. Opt for a gentle, hydrating cleanser that suits your skin type. For an extra boost, consider double cleansing in the evening—first with an oil-based cleanser to dissolve makeup, followed by a water-based cleanser to remove any residue. This two-step process can significantly enhance your skin's clarity and radiance.

Incorporating exfoliation into your routine is another vital step for achieving that Hollywood glow. Exfoliation helps to slough off dead skin cells, revealing a brighter and smoother complexion beneath. Hollywood stars often rely on chemical exfoliants, such as alpha-hydroxy acids (AHAs) or beta-hydroxy acids (BHAs), which can be more effective and less abrasive than physical scrubs. Aim to exfoliate two to three times a week, depending on your skin's sensitivity. Regular exfoliation not only improves skin texture but also allows subsequent products to penetrate more effectively, maximizing their benefits.

Hydration is key for maintaining a luminous complexion. Hollywood's top makeup artists often emphasize the importance of using a good moisturizer tailored to your skin type. Look for products that contain hyaluronic acid, which can hold up to 1,000 times its weight in water, providing intense hydration. Additionally, consider incorporating a facial oil into your routine, especially if you have dry or combination skin. Oils rich in vitamins and antioxidants can lock in moisture and create a dewy, healthy appearance that radiates from within.

Sunscreen is a non-negotiable step in any skincare regimen, particularly for those desiring a glowing complexion. Prolonged sun exposure can lead to uneven skin tone, hyperpigmentation, and premature aging, all of which detract from that sought-after glow. Choose a broad-spectrum sunscreen with at least SPF 30 and apply it daily, even on cloudy days. For added convenience, consider tinted sunscreens that provide a hint of color while still protecting against UV damage. This not only helps to shield your skin but also offers a subtle luminosity that can enhance your overall appearance.

Lastly, don't underestimate the power of nutrition and hydration from within. Many Hollywood stars swear by a balanced diet rich in antioxidants, vitamins, and healthy fats to maintain their radiant skin. Foods like avocados, berries, nuts, and leafy greens can have a significant impact on your skin's health. Additionally, staying hydrated by drinking plenty of water throughout the day helps to flush out toxins and keep your skin plump. Incorporating these dietary habits, along with a diligent skincare routine, can help you achieve that Hollywood glow that turns heads and leaves a lasting impression.